Copyright

Protected by copyright law.

No piece of this book might be replicated, conveyed, or communicated in any structure or using any and all means, including copying, recording, or other electronic or mechanical strategies, without the earlier composed authorization of the distributer, with the exception of brief citations epitomized in basic audits and certain other noncommercial purposes allowed by intellectual property regulation

Disclaimer

The data gave on this stage is to instructive and educational purposes as it were. It isn't expected as a substitute for proficient clinical counsel, conclusion, or treatment.
Continuously look for the counsel of your doctor or other qualified wellbeing supplier with any inquiries you might have in regards to an ailment. Never ignore proficient clinical guidance or postpone in looking for it in light of something you have perused on this stage.

Table of Contents

INTRODUCTION 1

DOSAGE 10

USES 17

SIDE EFFECTS 23

INTERACTION 26

PRECAUTION 46

FAQ 48

INTRODUCTION
Describe erythromycin.

Your doctor might advise taking erythromycin as a treatment if you have a bacterial infection. It's an antibiotic medication used to treat a variety of bacterial illnesses in adults and some kids. Similar to other macrolide antibiotics, it stops bacteria from growing and proliferating by interfering with their capacity to synthesizes proteins, all the while leaving human cells unaffected. Because Homophiles influenza and other bacteria are resistant to erythromycin on their own, erythromycin and sufficient dosages of sulfonamides must be used in conjunction to treat them.

Acute pelvic inflammatory disease, diphtheria, intestinal amebiasis, pertussis, syphilis, respiratory tract infections, and skin infections are just a few of the ailments that erythromycin is used to treat and prevent. In individuals who have experienced an allergic reaction to penicillin or sulfa medications, this medication is also used to prevent repeated episodes of rheumatic fever.

Erythromycin has long been used to treat a variety of respiratory diseases, including chlamydia, newborn conjunctivitis prevention, and community-acquired pneumonia and Legionnaires disease. Additionally, the FDA has approved it for the treatment of rheumatic fever, syphilis, intestinal amebiasis, prophylaxis, skin infections, and pelvic inflammatory disease (PID). Moreover, it works well to cure acne when combined with benzoyl peroxide or retinoic cream. This exercise will emphasize the pharmacology, adverse event profile, mechanism of action, and monitoring, pertinent interactions) that are important for interprofessional team members to be aware of while treating patients with infections and other diseases for which this medication is recommended.

The therapeutic efficacy of erythromycin, clarithromycin, and azithromycin in treating common respiratory and skin/skin-structure infections is demonstrated. Treatment for Chlamydia trachomatis-related cervicitis and no gonococcal urethritis is also efficacious with erythromycin and azithromycin. Clarithromycin and azithromycin have better tolerance than erythromycin. However, when it comes to pharmacokinetic parameters including tissue distribution, half-life, and drug interactions, clarithromycin is more comparable to erythromycin. It is common to misunderstand the distinctions between the azaleas (azithromycin) and macrolides (erythromycin and clarithromycin) with regard to their pharmacokinetics and pharmacodynamics, spectrum of activity, safety, and cost. Variations in tissue half-life, volume of distribution, intracellular: extracellular ratio, and in vivo potency are explained by the uptake and release of these chemicals by fibroblasts and white blood cells. Even while research on microbiology shows that gram-positive organisms are as vulnerable Azithromycin is far more effective against Homophiles influenzas isolates than either erythromycin or clarithromycin. When determining in vivo action against bacterial infections, concentrations attained at the infection site and duration above the minimum inhibitory concentration are equally significant as in vitro activity. The usage of these agents during pregnancy and their medication interactions vary, according to an analysis of safety data. Pharmacokinetic medication interactions between erythromycin and clarithromycin with theophylline, terfenadine, and carbamazepine are revealed by safety data analysis; these interactions are not observed with azithromycin. Pregnancy category B medications include azithromycin and erythromycin, while category C medications include clarithromycin. The careful selection of treatment for indicated illnesses can benefit from the many variations in erythromycin, clarithromycin, and azithromycin's pharmacokinetics, microbiology, safety, and cost.

The following are a few bacterial infections that are treated with erythromycin:

certain infections of the upper or lower respiratory tract
pneumonia brought on by Mycoplasma respiratory infection
some skin infections, such as whooping cough (*erythrism*) and listeria infection

Basics of erythromycin
There are two pill forms for erythromycin: immediate-release and delayed-release. "Immediate release" refers to a substance that enters your body instantly. "Delayed release" describes how the medication enters your body after going through your stomach.
Other types of erythromycin include an eye ointment, a topical gel, and swallow able

capsules. Additional forms of the medication are available, including erythromycin ethyl succinate (Retyped, E.E.S.). However, this article does not address these forms. Filipino scientist Abelard B. Aguilar sent some soil samples to his boss at Eli Lilly in 1949. Through the use of metabolic products, Aguilar was able to separate erythromycin from a strain of Streptomyces erythroid (later renamed Saccharopolyspora erythredema) that was present in the samples. Aguilar was not given any more recognition or money for his discovery.

A visit to the company's Indianapolis manufacturing factory was purportedly promised to the scientist, but it was never carried out. "A leave of absence is all I ask as I do not wish to sever my connection with a great company which has given me wonderful breaks in life," Aguilar stated in a letter to the president of the business. The request was turned down.

In 1993, Aguilar contacted Eli Lilly once more to obtain royalties. from medicine sales over time, with the goal of using them to establish a foundation for underprivileged and ill Filipinos. Additionally, this request was turned down. September of the same year marked his death. Lilly requested patent protection for the molecule, and in 1953, their request was approved.1952 saw the product's commercial debut under the name Liposome, which was derived from the Iloilo region of the Philippines, where it was first harvested. Ilotycin was another name for erythromycin in the past.

In an attempt to circumvent erythromycin's acid instability, researchers at Taisho Pharmaceutical, a Japanese pharmaceutical company, created the antibiotic clarithromycin in the 1970s.

Being a bacteriostatic antibiotic, erythromycin inhibits rather than kills germs in order to stop them from growing. Inhibiting protein synthesis is how this activity is carried out. Erythromycin inhibits the production of proteins by binding to the 23S ribosomal RNA molecule in the 50S subunit of the bacterial ribosome, which blocks the synthesis of peptide chains. Since humans lack the 50S subunit and only have the 40S and 60S subunits, erythromycin has no effect on the production of proteins in human tissues. Macrolide antibiotics function as immunomodulatory and anti-inflammatory drugs. Erythromycin prevented neutrophil infiltration in the periodontium and lungs in preclinical investigations. Erythromycin thereby provided protection against both inflammatory periodontal bone loss and deadly pulmonary inflammation. Moreover, because inflammatory conditions significantly lower the levels of developmental endothelial locus-1 (DEL-1) Erythromycin resistance can arise due to alteration of the 23S renal present in the 50S renal. The bacteria are able to continue producing proteins because the erythromycin is unable to attach to the ribosome. Erythromycin functions as a pro-motility medication in addition to a bacteriostatic macrolide antibiotic. It is an agonist for the hormone mottling, which promotes intestinal motility. bacterial via direct action), based on the kind of microorganism it is employed against and its concentration. Staphylococcus aureus, various Streptococcus species, Mycoplasma species, Legionella pneumophila (the bacteria that causes Legionnaire's disease), and Corynebacterium diphtheria (the diphtheria causative agent) are among the disease-causing pathogens susceptible to erythromycin.

The brand-name forms of erythromycin eyry-tab is another brand name for erythromycin delayed-release tablets. Currently, there isn't a brand-name version of erythromycin tablets with quick release available.

As erythromycin is a generic pharmaceutical, it is a precise replica of the active ingredient found in name-brand drugs. Eryn-tab is the brand name drug on which erythromycin is based.

It is believed that generic medications are just as safe and effective as the name-brand medications they replace. Generic medications are typically less expensive than name-brand medications.

Speak with your doctor if you have any questions about using Eryn-tab in place of erythromycin. Additionally, read this Health line article to find out more about the distinctions between name-brand and generic medications.

DOSAGE
What is the recommended dosage of erythromycin?

Your doctor will advise you on the appropriate amount to take. The following are typical dosages; however, you should always take the dosage that your doctor prescribes. Forms and strengths: Erythromycin is available in two forms: immediate-release tablets (250 mg and 500 mg), and delayed-release tablets (250 mg, 333 mg, and 500 mg). Both forms indicate that the medication is released into your body immediately, while the delayed-release tablets are released into your body after passing through your stomach.

suggested dosages

Erythromycin immediate-release tablet dose recommendations are 250 mg four times a day or 500 mg twice a day. In most cases, treatment lasts between six and fourteen days, but sometimes it lasts longer.

The precise number of days your erythromycin therapy will last will be discussed with you by your doctor. It's crucial that you take erythromycin for the entire prescribed duration, even if you begin to feel better before completing all of your doses, as prescribed by your doctor.

Divided into three or four distinct doses, the maximum suggested daily dose is 4,000 mg (e.g., 1,000 mg taken four times per day).

Adult dosage of tablets with delayed release

The dosages for erythromycin delayed-release pills and immediate-release tablets are interchangeable. outlined previously. However, 333 mg of this type should be taken every eight hours according to a prescription.

Children's dose of erythromycin

Children's erythromycin dose is based on a number of variables. These include the type and severity of the infection being treated, as well as the child's body weight in kilograms (kg). The appropriate dosage will be determined by your child's physician.

Children often receive three or four doses of 30 to 50 milligrams per kilogram (mg/kg) of erythromycin each day. A daily total of 4,000 mg is the maximum dosage.

In the case of a toddler weighing 33.2 kg (about 73 pounds), a physician would recommend 250 mg of erythromycin administered four times daily (a total of1,000 milligrams daily).
Rather to pills, erythromycin liquid suspensions are frequently given for children; however, that form is not covered in this article. Your child's physician can provide you with more information regarding the dosage if the liquid suspension is prescribed.

The toxic kinetics
Erythromycin's ester and ester salts are absorbed into the systemic circulation from the small intestine in varying amounts (18–45%). Overall, the formulation used to inject erythromycin determines its bioavailability; the base formulation has the least bioavailability, while the estimate salt (liposome brand) has

the highest bioavailability. The ethyl succinate salt's bioavailability varies greatly. While ethyl succinate salt is better absorbed when given with meals, most erythromycin formulations are more fully absorbed when given during a fast. Peak serum erythromycin concentrations vary, as would be expected, and depend on the formulation consumed. They typically occur 2-4 hours after delivery. Within one hour of the lactobionate or gluceptate salts being injected intravenously, peak plasma concentrations occur.

After entering with an estimated Vida of 0.6–0.7 l kg−1, erythromycin is broadly disseminated in the body through the systemic circulation. About 70–90% of the medication is linked to plasma proteins. Due to its extensive clinical use in treating intracellular infections, the majority of the medication is located in the intravascular area. The majority of the drug is eliminated through the bile, with only 5–10% of the drug being eliminated unaltered in the urine after substantial metabolism. The half-life of erythromycin is approximately two to three hours.

The substrate of the cytochrome P450 (CYP 450) 3A4 is enzyme is erythromycin. Erythromycin increases its own metabolism by demethylations and oxidizing to nitro alkane metabolites after it is linked to CYP 3A. The CYP 3A4 is enzyme's iron appears to form persistent complexes with these nitro alkane metabolites, reducing the enzyme's ability to operate. Depending on The cornerstone of erythromycin-associated metabolic-based drug-drug interactions is CYP 3A4 activity, which can be suppressed to undetectable activity depending on the dosage and duration of erythromycin medication.

Human Pharmacokinetics

Erythromycin's pharmacokinetics are different from those of the more recent macrolides in a number of respects. Acid inactivates erythromycin basic, which is absorbed from the digestive tract in varying amounts. When taking erythromycin on an empty stomach, the drug's serum levels rise. To get around these issues, several erythromycin strains that are resistant to acid have been created. The bioavailability of azithromycin, clarithromycin, and dirithromycin is higher than that of erythromycin due to their superior absorption and acid stability. All the macrolides are extensively dispersed around the body, with the exception of the central nervous system. The liver metabolizes these substances to differing extents based on the specific agent. In contrast to erythromycin and clarithromycin, azithromycin does not undergo significant metabolism. The pharmacokinetics of clarithromycin and azithromycin permit shorter dosage schedules due of extended tissue concentrations Enzed and Alvarez-Eldora (1999

The "broad spectrum treatment and control of bacterial disease" is another application of erythromycin in fish care. Fish bacterial infections such as body slime, mouth fungus, furunculosis, bacterial gill sickness, and hemorrhagic septicemia can all be managed and treated with this medication. Erythromycin is mostly used in fish care for treatments that target gram-positive bacteria.

USES

Many different types of bacterial infections are treated with erythromycin. Additionally, it can be used to stop some bacterial infections. One example of a macrolide antibiotic is erythromycin. It functions by halting bacterial growth. Only bacterial illnesses are treated or prevented by this antibiotic. For viral illnesses, like the flu or the common cold, it is ineffective. Any antibiotic that is used unnecessarily may stop working against subsequent illness The Streptococcus, Staphylococcus, Hemophilic, and Corynebacterium genera of bacteria that cause infections of the skin and upper respiratory tract can be treated with erythromycin. The MIC susceptibility information for a few important microorganisms for medicine is shown below.

Blood borne pathogen: 0.015 to 256 mg/ml
Phenotypic staphylococci: 0.023 to 1024 mg/ml
Pyogenesis streptococcus: 0.004–256 mg/ml
0.015 to 64 mg/ml of Corynebacterium minutissimum

Because of this promotility effect, it might be helpful in treating gastroparesis. It has been demonstrated to help severely sick patients with their eating intolerances. Additionally, intravenous erythromycin can be administered during endoscopy to help empty the stomach and improve endoscopic visibility, which could improve the accuracy of the diagnosis and the course of treatment.

In certain cases, erythromycin is also used to prevent heart infections in patients undergoing dentistry or other treatments. Discuss the potential hazards of taking this drug for your illness with your doctor. Before receiving dental procedures, patients with valvar abnormalities of the heart and those who are allergic to penicillin can use erythromycin to prevent infections of the heart's valves, known as endocarditis, and recurrent rheumatic fever.

Erythromycin Base Film tab (erythromycin tablets) should only be used to treat or prevent infections that are confirmed to be caused by susceptible bacteria or that are highly suspected to be so in order to prevent the emergence of drug-resistant bacteria and preserve the efficacy of these and other antibacterial medications. When choosing or altering an antibiotic therapy, culture and susceptibility data should be taken into account. Local epidemiology and susceptibility patterns may aid in the empirical therapy selection process in the lack of such data.

Diphtheria: infections caused by Corynebacterium diphtheria, which are treated with antitoxin in addition to eradicating the organism in carriers and preventing the development of carriers.

Erythrismal: For the management of Corynebacterium minutissimum infections.

Ent amoeba histolytic a-induced intestinal amebiasis (oral erythromycins alone). Other medications are needed to treat extra enteric amebiasis.

Neisseria gonorrhea-caused acute pelvic inflammatory disease: Erythrosine® Lactobionate-I.V. (erythromycin lactobionate for injection, USP) is an alternative medication used to treat N. gonorrhea-caused acute pelvic inflammatory disease in female patients who have previously shown penicillin sensitivity. It is followed by oral erythromycin base. Prior to starting erythromycin treatment for gonorrhea, patients should undergo a syphilis serologic test. Three months later, they should have a follow-up syphilis serologic test.

Treatment with erythromycins is recommended for the following illnesses brought on by Chlamydia trachomatis: pregnancy-related urogenital infections, neonatal conjunctivitis, and infantile pneumonia. Erythromycin is recommended for the treatment of individuals with simple Chlamydia trachomatis infections of the urethra, endocardial tract, or rectal tract when tetracycline are contraindicated or not tolerated.3

Erythromycin is recommended for the treatment of Urea plasma urealyticum-induced no gonococcal urethritis when tetracycline's are contraindicated or not tolerated.3.

Treponema pallidum is the cause of primary syphilis. For people allergic to penicillin's, erythromycin (oral forms only) is another therapy option for primary syphilis. Examining spinal fluid both prior to and throughout therapy are important aspects of managing primary syphilis.

Legionella pneumophila is the cause of legionnaires' disease. Despite the lack of controlled clinical efficacy research, in The limited first clinical data and in vitro evidence point to erythromycin's potential efficacy in treating Legionnaires' Disease.

Prevention

Prevention of Rheumatic Fever's Initial Attacks: According to the American Heart Association, penicillin is the best medication to treat Streptococcus pyogenic infections of the upper respiratory tract, such as tonsillitis or pharyngitis, in order to prevent rheumatic fever from occurring.3 Patients with penicillin allergies should be treated with erythromycin. Ten days should pass during the administration of the therapeutic dose.

Preventing Repeated Rheumatic Fever Attacks: The American Heart Association states that the best medications for preventing recurring episodes of rheumatic fever are either penicillin or sulfonamides. The recommended course of treatment for persons allergic to penicillin and sulfonamides is oral erythromycin. American Heart Association in streptococcal pharyngitis long-term prophylaxis (to prevent recurring attacks of rheumatic fever).

SIDE EFFECTS
What adverse effects does erythromycin have?
Erythromycin can have minor to severe adverse effects, just like most medications. Some of the most typical adverse effects that erythromycin may produce are listed in the lists below. Not every potential adverse effect is included in these lists.

Remember that a drug's negative effects can vary depending on:
your age, additional medical issues You also take additional drugs.

mild consequences

The moderate side effects that erythromycin might produce are listed below. Consult with your physician or pharmacist to find out about more mild side effects. The prescribing guidelines for erythromycin delayed-release and immediate-release tablets are also available for reading.

Among the mild erythromycin adverse effects that have been documented are:

feeling sick and throwing up

stomach ache

diarrhea decreased hunger

mild allergic response* Many medications' mild side effects can disappear in a few days to a few weeks. Consult your physician or pharmacist, nevertheless, if they start to cause you problems.

The following are serious erythromycin adverse effects that have been documented:
liver issues
heart rhythm issues, such as arrhythmia
pancreatitis (pancreatic edema) and long QT syndrome
seizures
interstitial nephritis, or kidney edema
reversible hearing loss colitis, or colon enlargement brought on by an infection with Clostridium difficile (or "C. diff")
severe allergic response

What is the purpose of erythromycin?
Adults and certain children are taken erythromycin to treat a variety of bacterial illnesses.
Examples of bacterial infections that can be treated with erythromycin include:

certain infections of the upper or lower respiratory tract

pneumonia brought on by Mycoplasma respiratory infection

a few skin conditions, such as erythrismal and listeria

the whooping cough, or pertussis

Moreover, in patients allergic to penicillin, erythromycin may be administered to prevent bouts of rheumatic fever. (Serious strep throat complications, such as rheumatic fever, are uncommon in the US but still common in some other countries.)

Erythromycin functions by preventing bacteria from producing the proteins they require to thrive. The bacteria that are causing your infection cannot proliferate without these proteins and will ultimately perish.

INTERACTION
Drug Interactions with Base Film tab Erythromycin

Increased serum theophylline levels and possible theophylline toxicity may result from the use of erythromycin in patients receiving high theophylline dosages. Theophylline dosages should be lowered while a patient is on concurrent erythromycin therapy in the event of theophylline toxicity and/or increased serum theophylline levels.

Digoxin serum levels have been found to be raised when erythromycin and digoxin are administered concurrently. When erythromycin and oral anticoagulants are taken together, there have been reports of enhanced anticoagulant effects. In older patients, erythromycin's interactions with oral anticoagulants may have more marked increased anticoagulation effects.

The cytochrome p450 enzyme system's 3A isoform subfamily is both a substrate and an inhibitor of erythromycin (CYP3A). Coordination of operations of erythromycin and a medication that is predominantly metabolized by CYP3A may be linked to increases in drug concentrations, which may intensify or extend the concurrent drug's beneficial and harmful effects. When patients are using erythromycin concurrently, dosage changes may be explored, and when practicable, close monitoring of the serum concentrations of medications largely metabolized by CYP3A is recommended.

Some examples of CYP3A-based medication interactions that are clinically relevant are included below. There may also be interactions with other medications that the CYP3A isoform metabolizes. In post-marketing experience, the CYP3A-based medication interactions listed below have been noted with erythromycin products:

Ergotamine/dihydroergotamine: In certain patients with acute ergot poisoning, characterized by severe peripheral vasospasm and dysesthesia, concurrent use of erythromycin and ergotamine or dihydroergotamine has been linked. Triazolobenzodiazepines and similar benzodiazepines, including triazolam and alprazolam: According to reports, erythromycin can make triazolam and midazolam less clear, which can enhance the benzodiazepine's pharmacologic effects.

HMG-CoA Reductase Inhibitors: It has been observed that erythromycin raises the concentrations of these drugs (lovastatin, simvastatin, etc.). Rhabdomyolysis has been observed in a small number of patients who are concurrently taking these medications.

Erythromycin has been shown to raise the systemic exposure (AUC) of sildenafil (Viagra). The dosage of sildenafil should be lowered. (See insert in Viagra packaging.)

Reports of unplanned or documented encounters involving CYP3A-based interactions of erythromycin combined with vinblastine, methylprednisolone, cilostazol, tacrolimus, alfentanil, disopyramide, cyclosporine, carbamazepine, and bromocriptine

It is not recommended to take erythromycin with cisapride, pimozide, astemizole, or terfenadine together. Refer to the CONTRAINDICATIONS.
Furthermore, erythromycin has been reported to interact with medications such as phenytoin, valproate, and hex barbital that are not believed to be metabolized by CYP3A. When used concurrently, erythromycin has been shown to dramatically affect the metabolism of astemizole and terfenadine, two no sedating antihistamines. There have been sporadic reports of severe cardiovascular side effects, including as torsade's de pointes, other ventricular arrhythmias, cardiac arrest, and electrocardiographic QT/QTcB interval lengthening. Refer to the CONTRAINDICATIONS. Furthermore, rare reports of mortality associated with concurrent erythromycin and terfenadine use have been

made.

When erythromycin and cisapride are taken together, there have been post-marketing reports of medication interactions that cause torsade de pointes, ventricular fibrillation, ventricular tachycardia, QT prolongation, and cardiac arrhythmias. Interactions between Drug and Laboratory Test: Erythromycin impedes urine catecholamine fluorometric measurement.

Reactions between medication and supplements

Many different types of medications can interact with erythromycin.

Because they interact with erythromycin, some medications should not be taken together. Among these medications are:

the statin medications lovastatin (Altered) and simvastatin (Zocor)

the headache medications pimozide (Oral) and ergotamine (Erg Omar) or dihydroergotamine (Migraine, Tracheas)

If your doctor advises it, using erythromycin with other medications may still be safe even when they interact with one another. Among them are:

the heart medication Diltiazem (Cardizem), amlodipine (Norvasc), or verapamil (Verulam, etc.)

the statin medication Actavist (atorvastatin)

the gout drug colchicine (Mitigare, Colcrys)

theophylline (also known as Theo-24)

blood thinner medications

Viagra's sildenafil

Not every kind of medication that could interact with erythromycin is included in this list. You can learn more about these interactions from your physician or pharmacist. :

... any other side effects that erythromycin use may have.

When combined with antiarrhythmic medications such as sotalol (Bet apace), amiodarone (Cordarone), berylliums (Braylon), disopyramide (nor pace), dovetailed (Tikosyn), procainamide (Presently), quinidine (Quinaglute, Quinines, Quinoas), and disopyramide (Nor pace), erythromycin amplifies the effects of these medications, potentially causing torsade's de pointes.

By enhancing the kidneys' ability to eliminate erythromycin, theophylline such theophylline (Theo-Dur), oxtriphylline (Choledyl SA), and aminophylline (Phyllocontin) lower blood levels of erythromycin and perhaps lessen its efficacy. On the other hand, erythromycin prevents the liver from breaking down theophylline's through metabolism, which raises the amounts of the drug in the blood. Seizures and irregular heartbeats are among the negative effects that might result from high theophylline levels. Consequently, theophylline dosage should be lowered or the amount of theophylline in the

Because erythromycin increases the risk of cardiac toxicity, including torsade's de pointes, ventricular tachycardia, and death, it should not be used in conjunction with astemizole or terfenadine. Erythromycin should also be used with caution when taking the following medications:

Alfentanil: Erythromycin may lessen plasma clearance and increase the amount of time the medication acts; Erythromycin has the ability to block carbamazepine and valproic acid, which increases medication concentration and toxicity; Digoxin: Erythromycin acts on the intestinal microbiota to make digoxin active, which raises the amount of digoxin in the blood; Erythromycin boosts the drug's impact and decreases its elimination when used with midazolam or triazolam. Erythromycin, in short, treats infections of the skin, eyes, or respiratory tract. The medication must be taken by patients exactly as recommended by the physician to guarantee patient safety and improve therapeutic efficacy.

Grapefruit and erythromycin can interact. It is not advised to consume grapefruits or grapefruit juice when taking erythromycin. By doing this, you may be more susceptible to adverse effects or your current side effects may worsen.

For patients suffering from gastroparesis, erythromycin is prescribed because of its strong promotility activity. After using erythromycin as a promotility agent for an extended period of time, the doctor should keep an eye out for the emergence of microbial resistance. Because of the possibility of an uncommon but catastrophic hepatic failure, liver function tests need to be monitored. Patients with cardiac issues or those on antiarrhythmic or interfering medications should be especially cautious as QT interval lengthening is a potential side effect. When a patient has severe diarrhea after taking erythromycin, the doctor should rule out pseudomembranous colitis, which has been linked to both mild and life-threatening cases.

Alerts

In some cases, erythromycin can have negative effects on individuals with specific medical conditions. The term "drug-condition interaction" refers to this. If erythromycin is a good course of treatment for you, it may also depend on other circumstances.

Before using erythromycin, discuss your medical history with your doctor. A few things to think about are listed below.

65 years of age or older. Adults 65 years of age and above are more susceptible to reversible hearing loss as an erythromycin adverse effect. If you fall into this age range and have a liver or kidney issue, your risk may be substantially higher.

Additionally, an uncommon but dangerous side effect of erythromycin is abnormal cardiac rhythm, which is more common in older persons. To find out more information regarding whether See your doctor to find out if taking erythromycin at your age is safe.

cardiac issues. Rarely, erythromycin may result in long QT syndrome and other heart rhythm issues. If you already have a cardiac condition, particularly if you have arrhythmia, your risk may be increased. Ask your doctor if erythromycin is a good option for you if you have a cardiac issue.

Insufficient magnesium or potassium levels. Erythromycin may, but infrequently, result in cardiac rhythm issues including long QT syndrome. If your blood already contains low amounts of magnesium or potassium, you may be more vulnerable. If using erythromycin is safe for you, your doctor will decide.

renal or liver issues. Erythromycin may result in liver or kidney damage. You could have a greater chance of experiencing these adverse effects if you currently have a real or liver issue. Additionally, using erythromycin may make your problem worse.

myasthenia grave. If you have myasthenia gravis, taking erythromycin may make your symptoms worse. Consult your doctor about the advantages and disadvantages of taking erythromycin if you have this illness.

If it is feasible, your doctor might treat your illness with a different antibiotic due to the risks.

seizures. Erythromycin users have had convulsions ever since the medication was made accessible for use. If you use erythromycin and have a seizure-inducing illness, such epilepsy, your risk of experiencing this adverse effect may increase.

an allergic response. If you've experienced Your doctor is unlikely to prescribe erythromycin if you have an adverse reaction to the medication or any of its constituents. Find out from them which other medications would be best for you.

Alcohol and erythromycin

It is advised that you abstain from alcohol when using erythromycin. This is because drinking alcohol may reduce the effectiveness of erythromycin in treating your infection.

Being pregnant and nursing

Generally speaking, taking erythromycin after the first trimester of pregnancy is safe. The first 12 weeks of pregnancy are referred to as the first trimester. Rare reports of infant cardiac defects have been made when this medication is administered during the first trimester. However, it's unclear for sure if erythromycin or other factors are to blame for this.

Small levels of erythromycin are passed into breast milk. Unless your doctor instructs otherwise, breastfeeding is generally regarded as safe while taking this medication. If you take erythromycin and nurse your child, keep an eye out for signs of irritation, diarrhea, and diaper rash in the infant.

How does one take erythromycin?
You will hear from your doctor about how to use erythromycin. They will also go over how often and how much to take. Make sure you adhere to your doctor's recommendations.

Utilizing erythromycin
Erythromycin is taken orally as a pill.

Labels and containers for medications that are easily accessible
Inform your doctor or pharmacist if you find it difficult to understand the label on your prescription. Medication labels that some pharmacies supply include:

feature braille, large print, and a code that can be scanned with a smartphone to convert the text to audio

Erythromycins A, B, C, and D are four closely similar chemicals that make up the majority of standard-grade erythromycin. These chemicals can differ by lot and can be present in different proportions. The most potent antibacterial agent was discovered to be erythromycin A, which was followed by erythromycin B. About half of erythromycin A's activity is possessed by erythromycins C and D. After being refined, a few of these related molecules are now ready for individual investigation and study.

macrolide

medication

Macrolides are a type of antibiotics distinguished by their enormous lactone ring structures and their ability to limit bacterial growth, or exhibit bacteriostatic properties. When erythromycin was extracted from the soil bacteria Streptomyces erythraeus in the 1950s, researchers made the initial discovery of the macrolides. Synthetic erythromycin derivatives, such as clarithromycin and azithromycin, were created in the 1970s and 1980s.

Although they can be given parenterally, macrolides are typically given orally. These medications are useful in treating penicillin-sensitive patients' streptococcus pneumonia and pharyngitis. They are used to treat pharyngeal carriers of the bacillus that causes diphtheria, Corynebacterium diphtherias, as well as pneumonias caused by either Mycoplasma species or Legionella pneumophila (the organism that causes Legionnaire illness).

Macrolides prevent the synthesis of bacterial proteins by attaching to a particular subunit of ribosomes, which are sites of protein synthesis, in sensitive bacteria. This effect prevents cell growth in the majority of species, but at high quantities, it can kill cells. Certain bacterial species, such as Staphylococcus aureus and Streptococcus pneumonia, have been shown to possess mutations that change the ribosomal subunit's macrolide binding site, making the bacterium resistant to the agents. Certain bacterial strains have also developed additional resistance mechanisms to macrolides, such as the activation of drug efflux proteins and the synthesis of enzymes that render drugs inactive.

Cephalosporin medication

Any of the β-lactam antibiotics known as cephalosporin prevent the formation of a structural element of the bacterial cell wall. Cephalosporium acre onium cultures were used to initially isolate the cephalosporin. Numerous derivatives with various antibacterial characteristics have been produced through modifications to the β-lactam ring, numbering over 20. When treating patients who are penicillin-sensitive, cephalosporin is frequently utilized as a substitute.
Roughly speaking, the cephalosporin's' activities have led to groupings. First-

generation cephalosporin's, such as cephalothin and cefazolin, are generally broad-spectrum antibiotics that work well against gram-positive and many gram-negative bacteria, such as many types of Escherichia coli and Staphylococcus and Streptococcus. They have also been utilized to combat Klebsiella pneumonias-related lung infections. In general, gram-negative bacterial species that have developed resistance to first-generation cephalosporin are more susceptible to the effects of second- and third-generation cephalosporin's, such as cefuroxime and cefamandole, and ceftazidime. The efficacy of second-generation cephalosporin's against gonorrhea, hemophilus influenza, and Bactericides' fragilis abscesses has been demonstrated. Many cephalosporin derivatives are useful in the treatment of meningitis because of their capacity to permeate the cerebral spinal fluid.

any bacterium belonging to the genus Mycoplasma, or the mycoplasma bacteria. Any species in the class Moll cutes or any genus in the order Mycoplasmas ales have also been referred to by the term Mycoplasma.

Among the tiniest bacterial species are mycoplasmas. The form of the cell varies from 0.3 to 0.8 micrometers [0.0000117 to 0.0000312 inch] spherical or pear to up to 150 micrometers [0.00585 inch] slender branched filament. The majority of Mycoplasma species are colonial, facultatively anaerobic microbes without cell walls. Among ruminants, carnivores, rodents, and humans, Mycoplasma species are parasites of the joints and mucous membranes lining the respiratory, genital, or digestive tracts. The bacterium produces toxic metabolites that build up in the tissues of the host and cause harm. M. pneumonia frequently but infrequently causes a deadly cases of pneumonia in people. A host's significant immunological response can also be triggered by a mycoplasma infection.

PRECAUTION
Inform your doctor or pharmacist if you have any allergies before taking erythromycin, including those to other macrolide antibiotics like azithromycin and clarithromycin as well as to any other medication. Inactive chemicals in this product have the potential to trigger allergic reactions or other issues. For further information, consult your pharmacist. Inform your doctor or pharmacist about all of your medical history before using this drug, including any instances of renal illness, liver disease, or myasthenia gravis.
QT prolongation is a heart rhythm disorder that erythromycin may aggravate. Rarely, QT prolongation can result in symptoms including acute dizziness and fainting, which require immediate medical attention, as well as a fast or irregular heartbeat that can be fatal.

If you take other medications that can cause QT prolongation or have certain medical conditions, your chance of developing QT prolongation may be higher. Inform your doctor or pharmacist about all the medications you take and if you have any of the following conditions before using erythromycin: a family history of specific cardiac conditions, sluggish heartbeat, QT prolongation in the EKG, and heart failure heart issues (sudden cardiac death, QT prolongation in the EKG). Additionally, low blood levels of magnesium or potassium can raise your risk of QT prolongation. If you take certain medications (such as diuretics or "water pills") or have health issues including extreme perspiration, diarrhea, or vomiting, your risk may go up. Consult your physician about the safe use of erythromycin.

In the absence of a confirmed or highly suspected bacterial infection or a preventive rationale, prescribing Erythromycin Base film tab (erythromycin tablets) is unlikely to benefit the patient and raises the possibility of the emergence of drug-resistant bacteria.

Patients with reduced hepatic function should use caution when administering erythromycin because it is mostly eliminated via the liver.

FAQ

Is pink eye treated with erythromycin eye ointment?

Indeed, pink eye and other bacterial eye infections can be treated with erythromycin eye ointment.

The topic of this essay is erythromycin pills. See your doctor for further information about erythromycin eye ointment's applications.

Can gastroparesis, sore throat, and acne be treated with erythromycin oral tablets?

It is not authorized to use erythromycin pills to treat gastroparesis, or delayed stomach emptying. Doctors may, however, continue to prescribe the medication off-label for this purpose. (Off-label use is when a doctor prescribes a medication for a use that is not authorized by the FDA.)

Many infections, including some that can be treated with erythromycin, are the cause of sore throats. However, the medication isn't meant to treat sore throats. It effectively addresses the illness causing your symptoms.

What is the difference between clindamycin and azithromycin and erythromycin?

Antibiotics such as clindamycin, azithromycin, and erythromycin are used to treat specific bacterial infections.

They are all offered as swallow able tablets,

but they can also be obtained in various forms. These medications also differ in a few other ways, such as how they cause various adverse effects. However, they can all result in diarrhea, especially severe diarrhea brought on by an infection with Clostridium difficile (or "C. diff").

Is erythromycin a penicillin-like drug?

Erythromycin is not a kind of penicillin, to be clear. Penicillin and erythromycin are examples of antibiotics. Yet erythromycin belongs to the class of antibiotics known as macrolides. Those who are allergic to penicillin's can utilize erythromycin. Your doctor can advise you on the appropriate use of erythromycin if you have a penicillin allergy.

I should provide Erythromycin when?

Usually, erythromycin is administered four times per day. Usually, this happens before breakfast in the morning, before lunch at around noon, before tea in the late afternoon, and before bed. These times should ideally be separated by at least three hours.

When should the medication begin to take effect?

After taking the medication for two to three days, your youngster ought to start feeling better. It is crucial that they take the prescribed medication for the entire recommended duration. Don't give up too soon.

And if my child gets ill and throws up?

Give your child the same dosage of erythromycin again if they become ill within thirty minutes of receiving it.
Don't give your child another dose of erythromycin if they become unwell more than half an hour after taking one. Await the subsequent regular dosage.

See your family physician, nurse, pharmacist, or hospital for advice if your kid becomes ill again. They will make a decision based on the particular medication involved and your child's condition.

Which antibiotic is erythromycin?

No. Erythromycin is not a drug that contains penicillin's. It's an antibiotic of a different kind called a macrolide. Your doctor may recommend erythromycin in place of penicillin-type medications if you have a penicillin allergy.

Is erythromycin safe to take when expecting?

The safety of erythromycin usage during pregnancy is unknown. According to animal research, erythromycin did not affect the fetus. If you are or want to become pregnant, speak with your healthcare professional. They can guarantee that erythromycin won't harm you or your unborn child.

For what number of days is erythromycin recommended?

The kind and severity of your infection will determine how long you take erythromycin for. While most infections may be cured in 7 days, certain infections may require up to 3 weeks to fully resolve. If you're unsure about how long you should take this medication, consult your healthcare professional and carefully follow the instructions on the label.

What distinguishes erythromycin from its ethyl succinate (EES) form?

While erythromycin ethyl succinate (EES) is available as a tablet or as an oral suspension, erythromycin is only accessible as a tablet. The body absorbs EES less readily than it does ordinary erythromycin. EES may possibly be more bearable than erythromycin due to its less adverse effects. Find out which one might be most effective for you by speaking with your healthcare professional.

Is erythromycin a treatment option for gastroparesis?

The FDA has not approved erythromycin for the treatment of gastroparesis, a disorder that causes the passage of food through the stomach to slow down or even stop. However, since erythromycin has been shown to accelerate the action of gut muscles, some medical professionals may short-term administer it off-label to treat gastroparesis. If you have any concerns about taking this drug for gastroparesis, consult your doctor.

The increasing availability of "omics" techniques has had a significant impact on the field of metabolic engineering of microbes for the purpose of producing useful chemicals on an industrial scale in recent times. Our systems-wide understanding of cell physiology, from transcriptional and translational regulation to morphogenesis, stress response, and many other processes in the cell, has significantly expanded thanks to the advances in genomics, transcript omics, proteomics, and metabolomics. The results of omics analyses have frequently inspired novel metabolic engineering strategies that have significantly improved the titres of industrially important metabolites like l-lysine, l-threonine, or xylitol particularly for production of metabolites with well-characterized biosynthetic pathways in well-known microbes. Furthermore, integrating various omics data types using systems biology techniques is a very promising tool in process development that will further expedite the creation of effective bioprocesses to produce both natural and artificial compounds.

Actinomycetes bacteria that live in the soil are very good at producing a wide range of physiologically active secondary metabolites, which are widely used in agriculture, animal medicine, and human health Antibiotics, antifungals, anti-cancer, immunosuppressive agents, insecticides, and other types of bioactive compounds with significant benefits to human health and the world economy are among these substances. These substances are created in trace amounts by bacterial cells as secondary metabolites that are not necessary in natural settings. The development of various strains and fermentation bioprocesses used to generate these metabolites on an industrial scale has been the focus of decades of research. The majority of the time, strains underwent rigorous strain selection with the goal of increasing target product yields after being randomly exposed to mutagenesis treatments [8, 9]. Thus, a number of strains currently in use in industry have significantly, enhanced secondary metabolite production by up to 1000 times. They also contain a large number of unidentified mutations that interfere with their regular developmental cycle, increase their sensitivity to environmental factors, and obstruct future efforts to optimize production.

It's obvious that omics techniques are creating new opportunities to quickly transform actinomycetes into highly developed and productive cell factories. Researchers will be able to specifically remove the metabolic bottlenecks of secondary metabolite biosynthesis without making unneeded or harmful alterations if they have a better grasp of their physiology. It has been suggested to use a "reverse engineering" strategy to identify production-critical variables by comparing wild strains to industrial high-producing strains created through random mutagenesis and selection.

Thanks to omics approaches, significant progress has already been made in understanding actinomycetes biology. For instance, actinomycetes strains' previously undiscovered capacity to synthesis a wide variety of distinct bioactive chemicals was discovered by genome sequencing. Nevertheless, the processes that lead to higher yields of valuable bioactive chemicals remain poorly understood, and the application of omics techniques to enhance the production of significant natural products at industrial scale has yielded only patchy results. There are probably a few explanations behind this: (1) The complex networks of global and pathway-specific regulatory genes and morphological differentiation found in actinomycetes' large genomes (up to 12 Map); (2) The intricate and poorly understood interrelationships between primary and secondary metabolic pathways during the bioprocess's production stage; (3) Laboratory media, where transcriptomic and In contrast to omics analyses in rich industrial media, which are hindered by challenges in isolating high-quality RNA and/or proteins, proteomic analyses are typically conducted and poorly reflect industrially relevant bioprocess conditions. (4) The majority of actinomycetes strains used in industry have probably been "over-mutagenized" during the strain improvement process, resulting in a large number of observed genomic variants (SNPs), many of which represent neutral or even negative mutations, which frequently result in morphologically and physiologically unstable strains that are hard to manage reproducibly in an industrial environment Compared to most other microorganisms, industrial actinomycetes present a greater challenge for the use of omics analysis and their interpretation because of all these features.

Saccharopolyspora erythraeus is a particularly intriguing organism to study since it is both a model representative of actinomycetes and the manufacturer of erythromycin, an antibiotic with great industrial and therapeutic value. Numerous research has examined the changes in gene expression that occur in both wild type and industrial strains of S. erythraeus during the bioprocess of erythromycin synthesis since the publication of the genome. Even with the advancements in these research, there is still much to be done to determine the functional significance of mutations discovered in industrial strains of S. erythraeus, pinpoint important mechanisms affecting erythromycin yield, and make sense of the relationships between erythromycin biosynthesis and other aspects of cellular metabolism. A deeper comprehension of these characteristics is crucial to permit the rapid increase of erythromycin output through metabolic engineering and synthetic biology techniques.

www.ingramcontent.com/pod-product-compliance
Lightning Source LLC
Chambersburg PA
CBHW071958210526
45479CB00003B/979